WORKBOOK TO ACCOMPANY

CAREER SUCCESS FOR HEALTH CARE PROFESSIONALS

DVD Series

Lee Haroun, EdD, MBA
Educator and Health Care Writer

Susan R. Royce, MS
Program Specialist and Curriculum Writer

THOMSON

DELMAR LEARNING

Australia   Canada   Mexico   Singapore   Spain   United Kingdom   United States

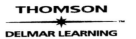

THOMSON

DELMAR LEARNING

Workbook to Accompany Career Success for Health Care Professionals
DVD Series
By Lee Haroun and Susan R. Royce

Vice President, Health Care Business Unit:
William Brottmiller

Editorial Director:
Cathy L. Esperti

Acquisitions Editor:
Marah Bellegarde

Developmental Editor:
Debra Flis

Editorial Assistant:
Jennifer McGovern

Marketing Director:
Jennifer McAvey

Marketing Coordinator:
Kim Duffy

Technology Project Manager:
Victoria Moore

Project Editor:
Jennifer Luck

Art & Design Specialist:
Christi DiNinni

Production Coordinator:
Jessica McNavich

ISBN 1-4018-3511-2

Contents

MCII

MCII

MCI

MCI

MCI

MCI

Introduction

You have chosen an exciting and challenging occupational area. Health care workers are needed more than ever, and this need is expected to grow in the future. An important part of your occupational training is learning technical skills such as taking a blood pressure, administering a breathing treatment, or filling out an insurance claim form. But there is much more to being a successful health care worker than mastering technical skills. In fact, skills such as listening and working well with others are just as important. Your future patients want someone who is understanding, listens well, and is respectful. Your future employers want someone who is dependable, cooperative, and ethical.

The *Career Success for Health Care Professionals DVD Series* contains interesting scenarios to help you learn and develop the nontechnical skills you will need on the job. The workbook contains activities and assignments you can use to apply what you learn from viewing the DVDs.

Patients who are unhappy with the way they are treated as people are much more likely to have doubts about the quality of care they are receiving. The DVD series and the activities in this workbook were designed to assist you to fully develop all the skills you will need to be successful in your chosen health care career. We hope you enjoy the DVD series and take advantage of the many opportunities provided to participate and increase your chances for future success.

LEARNING OBJECTIVES

1. Know your worth and importance as a health care worker
2. Be aware of the need to respect others as individuals of value
3. Understand empathy and its importance when working with patients
4. Learn to show respect and feel empathy for patients

GLOSSARY

assumption   Something that is taken for granted or thought to be a fact.

coding   Assigning numerical codes to information taken from medical records.

commitment   A promise to do something.

compassion   Feelings such as sympathy, caring, and love for others combined with a desire to help others.

culture   The values, shared beliefs and attitudes, social organizations, family and personal relationships, language, everyday activities, religious practices, and concepts of time and space of a given group of people.

diagnose   To identify or recognize a disease, based on observation, examination, and/or tests.

economic status   The amount of money a person earns and/or has.

empathy   Understanding another person's beliefs, feelings, and behavior (does not necessarily mean agreeing with them). Empathy should not be confused with sympathy, which means feeling sorry for someone.

ethnic background   One's race and culture.

heart murmur   A sound in the heart region that is different from normal heart sounds. A murmur may be caused by blood leaking through a heart valve that does not close properly.

innovation   Something new, such as a way of doing something or a piece of equipment.

insight   The ability to see and understand the inner nature of things.

insurance plans   In health care, plans in which people pay a certain amount each month to an insurance company. When they need health care, the insurance company pays an agreed-upon amount for their care.

preconception   Opinion formed before knowing and considering the facts.

vitals   (short for "vital signs") Measurements of blood pressure, temperature, pulse, and breathing rate. These provide information about how the body is functioning.

DISCUSSION QUESTIONS THAT APPEAR IN DVD 1

Scene 1

■ What kinds of personal things did Cleo discover about Mr. Jones?

_____

_____

■ How might this help her sessions with him?

_____

_____

■ How else might this contribute to the overall situation and to Mr. Jones's recovery?

_____

_____

Scene 2

■ How was David's behavior more respectful than Steve's?

_____

_____

■ What are some of the positive effects of David's respect for Carlos?

_____

_____

■ Was it appropriate for Dave and Steve to have their conversation in front of Carlos?

_____

_____

Scene 3

■ In what ways was Keisha unempathetic?

_____

_____

■ What could she have done to show more empathy?

_____

_____

■ How might this have changed the previous interaction?

_____

_____

Scene 4

■ What do you think of Dr. Osher's communication style?

_____

_____

■ How did Gwen demonstrate empathy?

_____

_____

_____

■ How did Gwen go beyond what was expected of her in this situation?

_____

_____

ADDITIONAL DISCUSSION QUESTIONS AND ESSAY PROMPTS

1. People who have health problems are often experiencing loss. How did loss affect each of the patients in this segment? What are some ways health care workers can help patients deal with loss? How do you think loss affects health? How do you think loss affects our ability to recover from health problems?

_____

_____

_____

_____

2. It is likely that many of your patients will be older people. What are some problems faced by aging adults? Do you think our society tends to discriminate against older people? Explain your answer. How can you contribute to the quality of life of your older patients? What can you gain from working with older people? Are there older people in your life who make a difference for you?

_____

_____

_____

3. "Most of us can work effectively with people who are pleasant. It takes special insight and caring to work with more challenging patients." Do you agree with this statement? What are some ways future health care workers can develop this "special insight and caring"?

_____

_____

_____

_____

4. What does it mean when we say that "every patient is an individual of worth"? Do you believe that all patients deserve the same care and consideration? How would you feel about helping a patient who has been convicted of a serious crime or is a drug addict and doesn't want your help?

_____

_____

_____

_____

5. The segment opened with a proverb: "He who has health has hope, and he who has hope has everything." What do you think this means? Do you agree with it? How important is health to you? Do you know anyone who has serious health problems? How do these problems affect his or her life?

_____

_____

_____

_____

6. Mr. Jones says that the physical therapy assistant helped him find the inner strength to try to use the walker. What do you think he meant by "inner strength"? How did Cleo encourage him? What are some other ways health care workers can help patients develop a positive attitude about their recovery?

_____

_____

_____

_____

7. David, the nurse who is caring for Carlos, the teen in the coma, says he believes that part of his job is to care for Carlos's mother. What do you think he means by this? Do you think health care workers should be concerned about families as well as their patients?

_____

_____

_____

_____

8. "Most of us take our view of the world for granted." Why is it often difficult for people to understand the views of others? What kinds of problems does this cause? What are some ways health care workers can learn about the views of their patients?

_____

_____

_____

_____

9. How is empathy different from sympathy? Why do you think empathy is more helpful than sympathy when working with patients?

_____
_____
_____
_____

CLASS ACTIVITIES

Class Activity Worksheet 1-1: Be Me

Think about each of the following patients and what their feelings, concerns, and needs might be.

1. Patient who is very hard of hearing and having difficulty understanding your questions
   Feelings: _____
   _____
   _____

   Concerns: _____
   _____
   _____

   Needs: _____
   _____
   _____

2. Patient who is frustrated because of wait for authorization from insurance company for an MRI to determine cause of neck pain
   Feelings: _____
   _____
   _____

   Concerns: _____
   _____
   _____

   Needs: _____
   _____
   _____

3. Patient who has just been diagnosed with cancer
   Feelings: _____
   _____
   _____

Concerns: _____
_____
_____

Needs: _____
_____
_____

4. Patient without medical insurance who comes to emergency room with very ill child

Feelings: _____
_____
_____

Concerns: _____
_____
_____

Needs: _____
_____
_____

5. Patient who is very overweight and seems hesitant to disrobe for exam

Feelings: _____
_____
_____

Concerns: _____
_____
_____

Needs: _____
_____
_____

6. Patient who appears to be in pain but is having difficulty communicating due to limited English

Feelings: _____
_____
_____

Concerns: _____
_____
_____

Needs: _____

_____

_____

Source: Adapted from Haroun, L., & Royce, S. (2004). *Teaching ideas & classroom activities for health care.* Clifton Park, NY: Thomson Delmar Learning.

Class Activity Worksheet 1-2: What Would It Be Like?

Consider how serious health problems and disabilities would change your life.

1. How might your life be different if you suffered from constant pain?

   _____

   _____

2. How would being blind affect your relationships with friends?

   _____

   _____

3. What kinds of extra help would you need and want if you were confined to a wheelchair?

   _____

   _____

4. How would you want to be treated if you had facial scars from being burned as a baby?

   _____

   _____

5. How would you hope to be treated by health care workers if you had to visit the hospital on a regular basis to receive therapy for a chronic health condition?

   _____

   _____

ASSIGNMENTS

Assignment 1-1: Understanding the Experience of Illness

Select one of the following diseases to research. Then answer the questions that follow.

1. Shingles (herpes zoster)—dealing with chronic, often severe pain
2. Osteoarthritis—swelling of joints, difficulty performing daily activities, pain; about 80 percent of all Americans are affected with this disease as they age
3. Fibromyalgia—chronic muscle pain, fatigue, headache, feelings of numbness and tingling, joint pain
4. Epilepsy—occasional seizures, ranging in severity
5. Cerebral palsy—spastic paralysis of the limbs, head rolling, difficulty with speech and swallowing; intelligence of patients with cerebral palsy is frequently normal or above average
6. Parkinson's disease—tremors, shuffling gait, muscular rigidity

7. Alzheimer's disease, early stage—difficulty remembering recently learned information, confusion, anxiety, poor judgment; the advanced symptoms do not come on suddenly, and many patients fully understand the future implications of the disease when they are first told of the diagnosis

8. Carpal tunnel syndrome—pain, muscle weakness, and tingling sensations of the hand

9. Ménière's disease—attacks of dizziness, nausea, and a ringing sensation in the ear that come without warning

10. Diabetes mellitus, type 1—daily insulin injections, controlled diet, possibility of hypoglycemia and hyperglycemia

11. Hemophilia—inability of the blood to clot normally; necessity of avoiding trauma, even small cuts, which can cause profuse bleeding

12. Emphysema—difficulty breathing and extreme fatigue

Worksheet for Assignment 1-1

Disease or condition selected: _____

Think about how having this disease or condition might affect your thoughts and daily activities.

1. Would there be limitations on what you could do, where you could go, and so on? If so, what are they? How would this affect the quality of your life?

   _____
   _____
   _____

2. Do you think that having this disease or condition would cause you to worry or be anxious? If yes, explain why.

   _____
   _____
   _____

3. Are there activities you enjoy now that you might not be able to do? If so, what are they? How might this affect the quality of your life?

   _____
   _____
   _____

4. Do you think your self-confidence would be affected by this disease or condition? If so, why?

   _____
   _____
   _____

Source: Adapted from Haroun, L., & Royce, S. (2004). *Teaching ideas & classroom activities for health care.* Clifton Park, NY: Thomson Delmar Learning.

Assignment 1-2: How You Make a Difference

"Regardless of your job title, you truly make a difference in the lives of others." List the contributions you can make in the health care career you plan to pursue. If you have not yet chosen a career, write about one in which you have an interest.

Worksheet for Assignment 1-2

Career: _____

Ways I can improve the lives of future patients:

1. _____
2. _____
3. _____
4. _____
5. _____
6. _____
7. _____
8 _____
9. _____
10. _____

Assignment 1-3: Developing Empathy in Your Everyday Life

Use the questions on the worksheet as prompts for thinking about how you can increase your empathy and apply it to the encounters you have with other people every day.

Worksheet for Assignment 1-3

1. What are some things I can do to better understand and respect the people I spend time with every day?

   _____

   _____

2. What are some things I can start doing to develop relationships with people I have either ignored or have had problems dealing with?

   _____

   _____

3. What can I do to be a better friend?

   _____

   _____

4. What can I do to be a better family member?

   _____

   _____

5. What can I do to become a better classmate?

_____

_____

6. How can I encourage others to do their best and achieve their goals?

_____

_____

7. How can I show others that I care about their well-being?

_____

_____

8. How can I be more understanding and accept differences in others, even when I don't agree with them?

_____

_____

Source: Adapted from Hwang, P. (2000). *Other-esteem: Meaningful life in a multicultural society.* New York: Brunner-Routledge.

Worksheet for Assignment 1-4: Exploring Your Feelings About Other People

Respecting others is an important characteristic of an effective health care worker. Fill in the sentences below to begin exploring your feelings about helping others.

One thing I value when helping others is _____

Helping other people makes me feel _____

When I meet someone I want to help, I _____

I want to be a health care worker who _____

I want to help others because _____

The way I would like other people to feel about me is _____

Worksheet for Assignment 1-5: Looking Beneath the Surface

Our actions can be the result of many causes. List as many explanations as possible for the following behaviors.

1. A friend who is usually glad to see you avoids you in the hallway at school.

_____

_____

_____

_____

2. You are a medical assistant. A patient who calls in to make an appointment is rude to you on the phone.

_____

_____

_____

_____

3. You are a nursing assistant. Your supervisor, who is usually pretty supportive, seems to be finding fault with just about everything you're doing today.

_____

_____

_____

_____

4. The medical biller in your office just doesn't seem to take her job seriously. She's been late to work three times in the last two weeks.

_____

_____

_____

_____

SUGGESTED TOPICS FOR WEB SEARCHES

Careers in health care

Comatose patients

Empathy

Health care beliefs of different cultures

The elderly: health changes, addressing their needs

Worksheet for Web Search

Topic: _____

Web address: _____

Sponsoring Organization: _____

What I learned: _____

_____

_____

_____

_____

How I might apply what I learned to my work in health care: _____

_____

_____

_____

_____

Name _____ Date _____ Class _____

PRETEST FOR CAREER SUCCESS DVD 1 *Cultural/Pt Sensitivity*

Select the answer that best completes the sentence, answers the question, or describes the situation.

1. Which of the following qualities is *most* important for health care workers to show respect for patients?

    a. sympathy

    b. empathy

    c. efficiency

    d. promptness

2. Accuracy when completing insurance claim forms

    a. may complicate the billing process.

    b. may cost the patient or practice more money.

    c. may help make the payment process hassle-free for the patient.

    d. is not important because insurance companies double-check the forms.

3. When dealing with difficult patients it is important to remember that

    a. the patient may be afraid and need some extra "hand-holding."

    b. the most important thing is to get the job done as efficiently as possible.

    c. you should focus on treating the illness rather than the patient.

    d. it is best to interact as little as possible.

4. On the health care team,

    a. all health care workers affect patients in important ways.

    b. medical billers have little to no effect on patients.

    c. only certain members of the team play an important part in the delivery of quality health care.

    d. only back-office personnel have much effect on patients.

5. The best way to deal with challenging patients is to

    a. leave their care to someone who has been trained to deal with challenging patients.

    b. hurry through your work so you can spend time with compliant patients who seem to want to get better.

    c. treat them with the same respect you show all your patients.

    d. let these patients know you are not happy with their behavior.

Choose T if the statement is true or F if the statement is false.

6. T F   When feeling empathy, you are feeling sorry for your patient.

7. T F   Learning what is important to patients can help you provide better health care.

8. T F   Sympathy is more important than empathy when working in the health care field.

9. T F   It is important to remember that your patient is a person, not a disease.

10. T F   Being familiar with other cultures can help you better serve your patients.

DISCUSSION QUESTIONS THAT APPEAR IN DVD 2

Scene 1

■ Nurse Garcia has an impact on the other characters. Describe her interactions with each one.

With Mrs. Anderson, the new resident:

_____

_____

With June, Mrs. Anderson's daughter:

_____

_____

With Sarah, the nursing assistant:

_____

_____

■ Nurse Garcia is the first link in a "chain of communication." Describe how this chain works.

_____

_____

_____

_____

_____

■ What methods did Sarah use to ensure that she understood the information given to her by Nurse Garcia?

_____

_____

■ How did this affect the care that the patient received?

_____

_____

Scene 2

■ Which components of active listening did Jen fail to use and with what result?

_____

_____

_____

■ Do you think Jen's remarks will influence Maria's decisions about smoking?

_____

_____

- How do preconceptions about others interfere with active listening?

_____

_____

Scene 4

- How do you think Sandy responded to the physician's comments?

_____

_____

- What do you think she said to the patient who approached her?

_____

_____

- Sandy says she is sorry. Does her body language convey that message?

_____

_____

- What message do Dr. Grier's nonverbal cues send to Sandy?

_____

_____

- Do you think the patient believes Sandy wants to help her?

_____

_____

- How did Sandy's nonverbal language send different messages than what she actually said?

_____

_____

- Look around the classroom. How are people using nonverbal cues right now?

_____

_____

ADDITIONAL DISCUSSION QUESTIONS AND ESSAY PROMPTS

1. Why are good communication techniques important when encouraging patients to adopt healthy lifestyle habits?

_____

_____

_____

_____

2. Explain why today's health care workers must be competent in providing effective patient education.

_____

_____

_____

_____

3. Why do you think Mrs. Anderson didn't tell Nurse Garcia that she couldn't hear her?

_____

_____

_____

_____

4. What clues did Nurse Garcia use to learn that Mrs. Anderson has a hearing loss?

_____

_____

_____

_____

5. What are some techniques to use when communicating with people who have hearing impairments?

_____

_____

_____

_____

6. What are some ways to improve your communication with people who have a limited knowledge of English?

_____

_____

_____

_____

7. Mrs. Anderson says that young people often speak to her as if she were an imbecile. Why do you think this happens?

_____

_____

_____

_____

8. Why do you think our society places so much emphasis on youth and appearance? What are the consequences for people of all ages?

_____

_____

_____

_____

9. Sarah, the nursing assistant, says she has learned that it is not up to the residents to entertain her, but, rather, it is up to her to help make their lives easier. What do you think of this statement? What are some ways health care workers can use communication to improve the lives of others?

_____

_____

_____

10. Is there someone you know who you feel really listens to you? What gives you that impression? Describe how you feel when you are with that person.

_____

_____

_____

11. "We don't always realize that listening and hearing are not the same thing." Explain what this statement means.

_____

_____

_____

12. How could Jen, the medical assistant, have helped Maria understand that smoking is a dangerous habit?

_____

_____

_____

13. How did the pharmacy technician use questions and feedback to better assist her customers?

_____

_____

_____

14. What are possible consequences of unclear communication with customers who are using drugs, both prescription and over the counter?

_____

_____

_____

15. In the last scene, Sandy's body language and tone of voice do not correspond to her words. Describe how Sandy's body language might have looked if it had matched her words when she said "I'm sorry" to the patient.

_____

_____

_____

_____

CLASS ACTIVITIES

Class Activity Worksheet 2-1: Giving Clear Messages

Describe the experience you had with your partner giving and receiving instructions.

1. How clear were your instructions? Was your partner able to understand everything you said?

_____

_____

2. How could you have improved your instructions?

_____

_____

3. How clear were your partner's instructions?

_____

_____

4. How could your partner's instructions have been improved?

_____

_____

5. Do you think poor listening is a problem for either of you? Explain why or why not.

_____

_____

6. Explain why clear communication is essential in health care.

_____

_____

_____

Class Activity 2-2: Overcoming Obstacles to Communication

Many things we say are very superficial and don't involve real communication. For example, automatically asking another student you see in the hall "How are you?" is usually more of a formality than a demonstration of real interest in the other person. Some communication exchanges are not only meaningless, they can be obstacles to further communication. The following chart contains several common verbal obstacles.

Verbal Obstacle	Example
Belittling or putting down the other person	Patient: I just can't seem to follow the diet that doctor gave me. Health Care Worker: You just need to use some willpower and stop eating so much!
Disagreeing without hearing the other person's point of view	Patient: I don't think the exercises the therapist gave me are doing me any good. Health Care Worker: Oh, sure they are. You're making good progress.
Giving advice that may not be helpful	Patient: My son seems to be getting sick a lot this year. Health Care Worker: You shouldn't let him eat so much junk food.
Defending yourself without considering the needs of the other person	Patient: I can't believe the amount of the bill I received from your office! I thought my insurance would cover the visit. Health Care Worker: Well, you probably didn't correctly fill out the paperwork we gave you.
Reassuring cliché that may not be true or sincere, but that sounds good to say	Patient: I'm so worried the treatment will be painful. Health Care Worker: Oh, it's not that bad. You'll be just fine.

Source: Adapted from Kalman, N., & Waughfield, C. G. (1993). *Mental health concepts* (3rd ed.). Clifton Park, NY: Thomson Delmar Learning.

Class Activity Worksheet 2-2: Overcoming Obstacles to Communication

Take turns with your partner responding to the following statements in a way that does not use a verbal obstacle.

1. I just know I'm going to flunk this class. I think the teacher hates me.

   _____

   _____

2. I'm really worried about my blood test. What if they find something really bad?

   _____

   _____

3. I wish I could lose some weight.

_____

_____

_____

4. I've put off writing the paper that's due next week. I'll never get it done on time.

_____

_____

_____

5. I've had these headaches for a long time. They'll never go away!

_____

_____

_____

6. It's my own dumb fault I broke my leg. I never should have tried skiing at my age.

_____

_____

_____

7. My father is having open-heart surgery. I'm really worried.

_____

_____

_____

8. I hate being in the hospital. I can't see what good it's doing me here.

_____

_____

_____

Class Activity Worksheet 2-3: Asking Helpful Questions

Working with a partner, use the following health care situations to practice asking questions. Your goals are to establish good communication and learn more about the other person. Take turns playing the parts of the health care worker and the patient. Include as many open-ended questions as possible. If this is a written assignment, use the space provided to write three questions for each situation.

Situation 1

You are a medical assistant. The patient is a young woman who is seeing the doctor for the first time. She says she is bothered by frequent headaches.

1. _____

2. _____

3. _____

Situation 2

You are a dental hygienist. The patient has come to see you at the insistence of his girlfriend. His teeth look like he's neglected them for years.

1. _____
2. _____
3. _____

Situation 3

You are a physical therapist assistant. The patient expresses dissatisfaction with the exercises the therapist has prescribed.

1. _____
2. _____
3. _____

Situation 4

You are a student in a patient care technician program. A fellow student is having trouble keeping up with the course work and is considering dropping out of the program.

1. _____
2. _____
3. _____

Situation 5

You are a pharmacy technician. A customer comes in with a prescription from the doctor but asks you to recommend something more "natural," such as an herb, that can be used instead.

1. _____
2. _____
3. _____

Class Activity Worksheet 2-4: Using Communication to Promote Understanding

1. Did you find it difficult to accurately summarize what the other person said? Explain why or why not.

   _____

   _____

2. Do you think the process improved your listening? Explain why or why not.

   _____

   _____

3. Did the process help you learn more about the other person's point of view? Explain why or why not.

   _____

   _____

4. How might you use feedback techniques to improve your communication with others?

_____

_____

Class Activity 2-5: It's in the Tone

Read each of the following sentences aloud and give the suggested meanings listed under each by changing the tone of your voice and the way you emphasize the words.

1. That's a good idea.
   - I like your idea.
   - That's really a stupid idea.
   - That's a really great idea and may help us solve a serious problem we're having.
2. Why did you do the procedure that way?
   - It looks like a good way and I'd like to know about it.
   - That seemed like a really dumb way to do it.
   - That was really time-consuming and I wish you hadn't done it that way.
3. I'd love to go the opera.
   - I like opera okay.
   - Are you kidding? I can't stand all that noise!
   - I love opera but can't afford the tickets. I can't believe you're willing to treat me.
4. What does he see in her?
   - She takes advantage of all the guys she dates. I'm worried he'll get hurt.
   - She's not very interesting. I wonder what they talk about.
   - She's so unfriendly. What does he find interesting about her?
5. I can't believe you're going out with him tomorrow.
   - Terrific news! You've liked him forever.
   - Are you kidding? He's rude and unfriendly.
   - You and I had plans. Are you going to dump our friendship because a guy asked you out?
6. How are you today?
   - I'm really interested in knowing.
   - You're always complaining. Let's get the negative report over with now.
   - I'm not really interested, but I'm being polite.

ASSIGNMENTS

Worksheet for Assignment 2-1: Better Listening Habits

1. What listening habit did you choose? _____

2. Were you able to focus attention on this habit during the time period assigned? Explain.

_____

3. Do you think you improved the quality of your communication? Explain why or why not.

_____

_____

Worksheet for Assignment 2-2: Worksheet Using Questions to Increase Understanding

One of the scenes shows Jen, a medical assistant, lecturing Maria about her recent decision to start smoking. Write five questions that Jen could have asked Maria that might have helped her better understand and help her. Include at least two open-ended questions.

1. _____
   _____?

2. _____
   _____?

3. _____
   _____?

4. _____
   _____?

5. _____
   _____?

Worksheet for Assignment 2-3: Nonverbal Communication

Research three forms of positive nonverbal communication, such as leaning forward to listen, and answer the questions for each one.

Example 1

Description of the nonverbal communication

_____

_____

How does it contribute to good communication?

_____

_____

How might a health care worker use this form of nonverbal communication?

_____

_____

Example 2

Description of the nonverbal communication

_____

_____

How does it contribute to good communication

_____

_____

How might a health care worker use this form of nonverbal communication?

_____

_____

Example 3

Description of the nonverbal communication

_____

_____

How does it contribute to good communication?

_____

_____

How might a health care worker use this form of nonverbal communication?

_____

_____

Assignment 2-4: Using Questions and Feedback

Over a three-day period, make an effort to use questions and feedback, as appropriate, in your daily communication. Then write a short paper in which you give examples of your questions and feedback techniques. Discuss whether you think using these questions and feedback improved the quality of your communication encounters.

Worksheet for Assignment 2-5: Communication in the Health Care Setting

List at least ten ways the nursing staff can use communication to help Mrs. Anderson (first scene) feel more comfortable and adjust to her new surroundings. Include suggestions for using questions and feedback.

1. _____

2. _____

3. _____

4. _____

5. _____

6. _____

7. _____

8. _____

9. _____

10. _____

SUGGESTED TOPICS FOR WEB SEARCHES

Active listening

Nonverbal communication

Patient education

Therapeutic communication

Wellness habits

Worksheet for Web Search

Topic: _____

Web address: _____

Sponsoring organization: _____

What I learned: _____

_____

_____

_____

_____

How I might apply what I learned to my work in health care: _____

_____

_____

_____

_____

Name _____ Date _____ Class _____

PRETEST FOR CAREER SUCCESS DVD 2

Select the answer that best completes the sentence, answers the question, or describes the situation.

1. When you communicate, the strongest message likely to get across to the listener is
   a. your verbal communication.
   b. your nonverbal communication.

2. Verbal communication consists of
   a. words and facial expressions.
   b. the way we hold our bodies.
   c. the words we speak.
   d. the words we read.

3. Nonverbal communication consists of
   a. our thoughts.
   b. our posture and gestures.
   c. the words we speak.
   d. our written communication.

4. Active listening
   a. is the same as hearing what the person said.
   b. is easy. We do it all the time.
   c. takes effort and practice.
   d. is something we are born knowing how to do.

5. Feedback has four forms:
   a. closed-ended, probing, restatement, and paraphrase
   b. restatement, paraphrase, clarification, and examples
   c. closed-ended, open-ended, probing, and leading
   d. probing, leading, examples, and paraphrase

Circle T if the statement is true or F if the statement is false.

6. T F Most people are born with good active listening skills.

7. T F Oral communication techniques include sending clear messages, asking useful questions, and requesting feedback.

8. T F Good active listening requires that you interrupt periodically so that you can clarify what is being said.

9. T F The words someone says are more important than the message being sent through his or her body language.

10. T F Good communication skills are often taken for granted.

Name _____ Date _____ Class _____

POSTTEST FOR CAREER SUCCESS DVD 2

Select the answer that best completes the sentence, answers the question, or describes the situation.

1. Which is the best description of active listening?

    a. using facial expressions to show our feelings while we listen

    b. using movement to show that we are listening

    c. establishing good eye contact

    d. hearing both the words of the speaker and the meaning and feelings behind the words

2. Have you been a patient here before? is an example of a(n)

    a. closed-ended question.

    b. open-ended question.

    c. probing question.

    d. leading question.

3. Are you taking your medication one hour before you eat? is an example of a(n)

    a. closed-ended question.

    b. open-ended question.

    c. probing question.

    d. leading question.

4. Are you taking a brand or generic form of your heart medication? is an example of a(n)

    a. closed-ended question.

    b. open-ended question.

    c. probing question.

    d. leading question.

5. What brings you to see the doctor today? is an example of a(n)

    a. closed-ended question.

    b. open-ended question.

    c. probing question.

    d. leading question.

6. For good active listening, you should

    a. carefully judge what the speaker is saying.

    b. think ahead to how you will respond.

    c. encourage the speaker with affirmative remarks.

    d. interrupt to clarify what the speaker is saying.

7. Providing feedback

    a. includes restatement, paraphrase, clarification, and examples.

    b. is only important when having a discussion of a medical nature.

    c. should be used with every conversation.

    d. is none of the above.

8. To give the speaker an indication that you are listening to her talk about a health problem, you should

    a. sit back in your chair.

    b. interrupt every now and then to repeat what the speaker is saying.

    c. respond by describing a similar problem you have had.

    d. nod your head and give occasional affirmative remarks such as "go on" or "okay."

9. Good oral communication technique includes

    a. answering questions quickly.

    b. sending clear messages, asking useful questions, and requesting feedback to ensure understanding.

    c. constantly thinking ahead to how you will answer.

    d. making sure both you and the speaker spend equal time talking.

10. Communication is

    a. getting your message across.

    b. hearing the speaker's message.

    c. a two-way process.

    d. none of the above.

Circle T if the statement is true or F if the statement is false.

11. T F   Feedback should be used throughout every conversation you have.

12. T F   Good communication includes verbal and nonverbal communication.

13. T F   A probing question requires a long response.

14. T F   An open-ended question is answered with one word.

15. T F   A leading question includes a possible answer.

Choosing from the list, write the word that corresponds to each definition.

accommodate	active listening	affirmative
chronic	clarification	closed-ended question
communication	empathy	feedback
imbecile	inadequate	leading question
open-ended question	paraphrase	perspective
probing question	restatement	

_____ 16. Understanding another person's beliefs, feelings, and behavior (does not necessarily mean agreeing with them)

_____ 17. A communication technique used to clarify and confirm what you hear

_____ 18. To adjust to something

_____ 19. A question that encourages a specific answer from the listener

_____ 20. Hearing the words of the speaker and the meaning and feelings behind the words

_____ 21. Sending and receiving a message

_____ 22. Positive

_____ 23. Repeating something as you heard it

_____ 24. Something or someone who does not meet set standards

_____ 25. Continuing, not acute or sudden

_____ 26. A question that encourages the listener to give a detailed explanation

_____ 27. A way of looking at things

_____ 28. Restate what you heard in your own words

_____ 29. Someone who is not very smart

_____ 30. Making clear; when listening, asking questions to be sure you understood what you heard

_____ 31. A question that encourages a simple answer such as "yes" or "no"

_____ 32. A question that requests additional information or clarification

LEARNING OBJECTIVES

1. Understand the importance of learning to think like a health care worker
2. Develop the thinking skills you will need on the job
3. Create an organized approach to identifying and solving problems

GLOSSARY

acute Severe, serious, of short duration.

apical pulse Measured by listening to the heart rate with a stethoscope.

consequence The outcome of an action or inaction.

critical thinking Purposeful thinking in which you observe, ask questions, distinguish facts from opinions, and apply what you have learned to new situations.

evaluate To judge or determine value.

instinct A biological impulse to act in a certain way.

malfunctioning Broken, not working correctly.

methodical Being orderly, symmetrical.

radial pulse Measured by feeling the surge of blood at the wrist.

reimburse To pay for expenses or services provided.

DISCUSSION QUESTIONS THAT APPEAR IN DVD 3

Scenes 1, 2, and 3

■ What did Mr. Jones say that gives clues about his condition?

_____

_____

■ What should the health care worker have considered when Mr. Jones said he was too warm?

_____

_____

■ Dee remarked that the patient's doctor should notice his symptoms. Is this a reasonable explanation for her failure to observe them?

_____

_____

■ How did Mark demonstrate that he was thinking on the job?

_____

_____

■ Was it Mark's responsibility to report what he thought might be an error?

_____

_____

■ How did Sandy demonstrate good thinking skills?

_____

_____

■ Why is it important for health care workers to take the time to think through what they do?

_____

_____

Scenes 4 and 5

■ Was Mandy right to call her supervisor?

_____

_____

■ Do you think she should have let the patient proceed with surgery because he had already waited so long for the approval?

_____

_____

■ How did Hal demonstrate that he was thinking like a health care worker in this situation?

_____

_____

Scene 6

■ How did Ms. Jameson's system help Karen find a solution to her eldercare problem?

_____

_____

ADDITIONAL DISCUSSION QUESTIONS AND ESSAY PROMPTS

1. Dee, the health care worker who doesn't question the heart patient's condition, says that doctors should be responsible for knowing about the condition of their patients. Why doesn't her assumption make sense?

_____

_____

_____

2. "Health care workers must learn to look at the big picture and think about the circumstances being presented to them." What does this mean? Why is it important?

_____

_____

_____

_____

3. What are some health care jobs in addition to medical biller that don't involve direct patient contact, but require attention and thought to avoid negative consequences for patients?

_____

_____

_____

_____

4. In three of the scenes, health care workers notified their supervisors when something didn't seem right. What types of situations should be reported to supervisors?

_____

_____

_____

_____

5. Do you agree with Mark that not following through to check on a possible error is the same as if he had made the error in the first place? Explain why or why not.

_____

_____

_____

_____

6. If you believe a superior's orders should be questioned, what is the best way to question those orders?

_____

_____

_____

_____

7. How does reporting errors you find contribute to providing quality service to all patients?

_____

_____

_____

_____

8. Health care workers are often in a hurry. What are some ways they can be both efficient and aware at the same time?

_____

_____

_____

_____

9. One of the components of critical thinking in health care is to "follow though on all your actions." What does this mean?

_____

_____

_____

_____

10. Mandy says she takes pride in her job. What does she mean when she says she trusts her instincts?

_____

_____

_____

_____

11. Dee tells Hal, the nurse who is to perform the finger stick, that he is making extra work for himself. Explain why you agree or disagree with her opinion of the situation.

_____

_____

_____

_____

12. In the beginning of the last scene, Karen needs help identifying her real problem. Why is it often difficult to see problems clearly?

_____

_____

_____

_____

13. What does it mean to take responsibility for your problems?

_____

_____

_____

_____

14. Some students who have many responsibilities get overwhelmed and don't finish school. How can they use problem-solving skills to improve their chances of completing their education?

_____

_____

_____

_____

CLASS ACTIVITIES

Class Activity Worksheet 3-1: Getting to the Heart of the Problem

In the scene with Karen and Ms. Jameson, Karen believes her problem is her ill father. In fact, her real problem is finding ways to care for her father's needs and complete her externship. Identifying the "real" problem is not always easy. In your group, discuss what you think might be the underlying problem in each of the following cases.

■ Emily believes her parents are "ruining her life" and preventing her from attending nursing school by their refusal to pay the entire cost of the tuition for her.

Are Emily's parents the problem? _____

If not, what might be? _____

■ Madison believes her supervisor, who has little time to answer questions, is to blame for the mistakes Madison has been making when she inputs data from medical charts onto insurance claim forms.

Is Madison's supervisor the problem? _____

If not, what might be? _____

_____

■ Roberto is a physical therapist assistant. His supervisor is concerned about the lack of progress shown by many of the patients with whom Roberto works. Roberto thinks that most of his patients aren't very motivated to get better.

Are Roberto's patients the problem? _____

If not, what might be? _____

_____

■ Greg, a medical assistant in a busy downtown clinic, feels intimidated by the physicians. He believes he could do a better job with the patients if the doctors didn't make him so nervous.

Are the physicians the problem? _____

If not, what might be? _____

_____

Source: Adapted from Haroun, L., & Royce, S. (2004). *Teaching ideas & classroom activities for health care.* Clifton Park, NY: Thomson Delmar Learning.

Class Activity Worksheet 3-2: Brainstorming Solutions

Once a problem is identified, the next step is to gather information and come up with possible solutions. In your group, come up with at least five possible solutions for the problems from Class Activity 3-1.

■ What are five ways Emily might finance nursing school?

1. _____
2. _____
3. _____
4. _____
5. _____

■ What are five actions Madison can take to reduce the number of errors she makes when inputting data on insurance claim forms?

1. _____
2. _____
3. _____
4. _____
5. _____

■ What are five things Roberto might examine to see if they are interfering with the progress of his patients?

1. _____
2. _____
3. _____
4. _____
5. _____

■ What are five things Greg can do to increase his self-confidence and ability to interact with the physicians?

1. _____
2. _____
3. _____
4. _____
5. _____

ASSIGNMENTS

Worksheet for Assignment 3-1: What Might Have Happened?

The following situations are based on the scenes in DVD 3. Think about the alternative situations presented here and answer the questions for each.

Suppose that Mark submitted the bill as he received it without question. What might have been the consequences for the facility in which he works? For Claire, his supervisor? For Miss Dawkins, the patient?

_____

_____

_____

_____

What might have been the consequences for Mr. Simmons if Sandy, the medical assistant, had not asked for the nurse's help in assessing his condition, but had simply sent him home?

_____

_____

_____

_____

Suppose that Dr. Mason checks Mr. Chadwick and determines he has pneumonia. What might have happened if Mandy had not notified her supervisor and no one else had noticed his symptoms?

_____

_____

_____

_____

What might have happened to Karen's future if she hadn't received help from Ms. Jameson? What might have been the impact on her self-esteem? Her financial situation? Her ability to help her ill father?

_____

_____

_____

_____

Worksheet for Assignment 3-2: The ABCs of Critical Thinking

Think about the actions of the characters in the scenes. Then list examples of actions you saw, both positive and negative, that relate to the following components of critical thinking.

1. Ask questions to gather needed information.

_____

_____

_____

2. Be aware and pay attention to what is going on around you.

_____

_____

_____

3. Compare what you observe with what you have learned.

_____

_____

_____

4. Don't take anything for granted. If something doesn't seem right, check it out.

_____

_____

_____

5. Evaluate situations and report them when appropriate.

_____

_____

_____

6. Follow through on all your actions.

_____

_____

_____

7. Get help when you are unsure of something.

_____

_____

_____

Worksheet for Assignment 3-3: Using the Five-Step Problem-Solving Process

Try using the five-step problem-solving process for yourself. Choose a problem you'd like to take care of and go through the process to see how it works.

1. Identify the Problem

   State the problem as clearly as possible. Taking responsibility for the problem enables you to start seeking a solution. The problem I want to solve is _____

_____

2. Gather Information

What I need to know is _____

_____

Sources of the information I need are _____

_____

_____

Summary of what I found out: _____

_____

_____

3. Create Alternative Solutions

Think of at least five alternative solutions.

1. _____

2. _____

3. _____

4. _____

5. _____

4. Choose a Solution and Put It into Action

Write the alternative you want to try first. _____

Explain how you will put it into action. _____

_____

_____

5. Evaluate and Revise (if necessary)

Describe how the solution you chose worked out. _____

_____

Do you need to try something else? If so, explain your revised plan. _____

_____

_____

SUGGESTED TOPICS FOR WEB SEARCHES

Critical thinking

Decision making

Medical mistakes

Problem solving

Professional responsibility

Worksheet for Web Search

Topic: _____

Web address: _____

Sponsoring organization: _____

What I learned: _____

_____

_____

_____

_____

How I might apply what I learned to my work in health care: _____

_____

_____

_____

_____

Name _____ Date _____ Class _____

PRETEST FOR CAREER SUCCESS DVD 3

Select the answer that best completes the sentence, answers the question, or describes the situation.

1. It is important for health care workers to look at the big picture because

    a. most supervisors don't have the time.

    b. only mistakes made in jobs with direct patient contact can have serious consequences.

    c. they may help a patient avoid a potentially dangerous situation.

    d. it helps keep their minds active and fresh.

2. The first four rules of the ABCs of thinking are

    a. ask questions, be aware, compare, and don't take anything for granted.

    b. ask questions, be quiet, compare, and don't take anything for granted.

    c. analyze, be aware, compare, and don't take anything for granted.

    d. analyze, be quiet, consider, and deliver results.

3. When you follow the five steps to problem solving, but the problem is not resolved, you should

    a. go through the steps again.

    b. give up. You won't find a solution that will work for you.

    c. ask someone else for help.

    d. evaluate and revise your original solution.

4. The first step to solving a problem is to

    a. ask someone for help.

    b. identify the problem.

    c. gather information.

    d. create alternative solutions.

5. Critical thinking is

    a. looking beyond the obvious.

    b. looking at something with a negative attitude.

    c. automatically reacting to an emergency without thought.

    d. being judgmental in new situations.

Circle T if the statement is true or F if the statement is false.

6. T F It is important for health care workers to thoroughly examine every situation before taking action.

7. T F It is important to always follow the doctor's orders without question.

8. T F Analyzing is the first step of the ABCs of thinking.

9. T F The last step to problem solving is to evaluate the results.

10. T F Since it is not appropriate for nonphysician health care workers to diagnose patients, they do not have to use critical thinking skills.

Name _____ Date _____ Class _____

POSTTEST FOR CAREER SUCCESS DVD 3

Select the answer that best completes the sentence, answers the question, or describes the situation.

1. Thinking like a health care worker means
   a. never questioning the doctor's orders.
   b. letting the patient know what you think his diagnosis might be.
   c. discussing patient care with coworkers.
   d. that you thoroughly examine every situation before taking action.

2. In the first scene when the patient said he was too warm and needed air, the health care worker should have
   a. opened the window as requested and gone to answer other patient calls.
   b. reported to a supervisor or physician that the patient was not feeling well.
   c. left the window closed because it was cold outside.
   d. told the patient that she thought he was probably running a fever.

3. Looking at the big picture and considering all the facts is important because
   a. other members of the health care team will pay attention to the details.
   b. you may help a patient avoid a complication or problem.
   c. other members of the health care team are too busy to pay attention to the big picture.
   d. it keeps you interested in your job.

4. The problem when Sandy took Mr. Simmons's pulse was that
   a. she could not detect a pulse.
   b. she was not properly trained to take a pulse.
   c. Mr. Simmons had a possible heart problem and needed to be checked by the doctor.
   d. she did not have confidence in her ability to take an accurate pulse.

5. The first skill in the ABCs of Critical Thinking is
   a. ask questions.
   b. analyze.
   c. anticipate.
   d. allocate.

6. Your school has a strict attendance policy and you know if you miss one more day, you will be dropped from your program. On Saturday, your car breaks down and you don't know how you will get to class on Monday. To solve this problem, you
   a. worry all weekend, but don't manage to get to school on Monday.
   b. try calling your instructor to see if the rule can be "bent" for you so you won't get dropped.
   c. identify your problem, gather information about your options, and decide your best solution is to carpool with a friend until you can afford to have your car fixed.
   d. check out the bus route, but decide you won't make it to class on time because the bus will take over two hours to get you there.

7. In the scene in which Mandy calls her supervisor regarding Mr. Chadwick's coughing, she should have
    a. checked Mr. Chadwick in and let the rest of the staff deal with his symptoms.
    b. called her supervisor without saying anything to Mr. Chadwick.
    c. handled the situation exactly as she did.
    d. checked Mr. Chadwick's vital signs before reporting his symptoms.

8. When Hal reported to the doctor that Mrs. Campbell had eaten prior to her finger stick,
    a. he had thought through what he was asked to do and the possible outcome.
    b. he was trying to make a diagnosis, something not appropriate for his position.
    c. he just made extra work for himself.
    d. he stepped out of line because he should have left it up to the doctor to know when patients are fed breakfast.

9. To effectively use your critical thinking skills,
    a. you should check with your supervisor each time you make a decision about patient care.
    b. you must be very smart.
    c. it is important to do your job without question.
    d. it is important to know the material necessary to carry out the duties of your position.

10. Critical thinking and problem-solving skills are important,
    a. but when the clinic is understaffed and you are extra busy, you should just do your job as quickly as possible without question.
    b. but only for doctors and high-level staff members.
    c. no matter what is happening around you.
    d. but only in emergency situations.

Circle T if the statement is true or F if the statement is false.

11. T F The first three steps of the ABCs of Critical Thinking are Analyze, Be aware, and Compare.

12. T F If your chosen solution to a problem does not work out, you should evaluate and revise your solution.

13. T F As a health care professional, you should never question a physician's orders.

14. T F You should be careful about critical thinking skills because they make you judge others.

15. T F Evaluating situations and reporting them when appropriate is an important part of critical thinking.

Choosing from the list, write the word that corresponds to each definition.

acute	apical pulse	consequence
critical thinking	evaluate	instinct
malfunctioning	methodical	radial pulse
reimburse		

_____ 16. The outcome of an action or inaction

_____ 17. To pay for expenses or services provided

_____ 18. Being orderly, symmetrical

_____ 19. A biological impulse to act in a certain way

_____ 20. Purposeful thinking in which you observe, ask questions, distinguish facts from opinions, and apply what you have learned to new situations

_____ 21. Severe, serious, of short duration

_____ 22. To judge or determine value

_____ 23. Measured by listening to the heart rate with a stethoscope

_____ 24. Measured by feeling the surge of blood at the wrist

LEARNING OBJECTIVES

1. Understand what it means to "do the right thing" in the health care setting
2. Know how health care workers apply ethics on the job
3. Learn to monitor your actions to avoid unethical actions

GLOSSARY

accountability   Responsibility.
ampule   A small, sealed container holding a liquid.
compromising   Weakening or giving up something.
condescending   Treating someone without regard for his or her dignity.
confidentiality   Not sharing information.
curt   Short or brief.
immense   Very large.
integrity   Doing what is right and honest.
professional ethics   A set of principles that guides a group's decision making regarding what is right and wrong.

DISCUSSION QUESTIONS THAT APPEAR IN DVD 4

Scenes 1 and 2

■ What was Mandy's ethical dilemma?

_____

_____

■ Did Mandy do the right thing? Why?

_____

_____

■ Did Keisha make the right decision in going to the nurse for help with the procedure?

_____

_____

■ What might have been the consequences if she had tried to perform the procedure herself?

_____

_____

Scenes 3 and 4

- How do professional ethics apply to the actions of the health care workers in the previous scene?

_____

_____

- What were the consequences of these actions?

_____

_____

Scene 5

- What exactly was Eileen's mistake?

_____

_____

- What could she have done to ensure that she did not make such mistakes?

_____

_____

ADDITIONAL DISCUSSION QUESTIONS AND ESSAY PROMPTS

1. "The right choice for a health care worker to make is not always the obvious one." Explain what this means and give an example.

_____

_____

_____

_____

2. Why is patient confidentiality such an important issue?

_____

_____

_____

_____

3. Where can health care workers learn about their scope of practice?

_____

_____

_____

_____

4. Where can health care workers obtain the code of ethics for their profession?

_____

_____

_____

_____

5. Two nurses in the scene in the busy clinic disagree about the proper way to give an injection. Comment on the way the younger nurse pointed out what she believed to be the more experienced nurse's error.

_____

_____

_____

_____

6. Do you agree or disagree with the worker in the busy clinic who believes it's not her job to do extra work when other employees don't show up?

_____

_____

_____

_____

7. How could good teamwork have helped improve the delivery of patient care at the busy clinic?

_____

_____

_____

_____

8. At the staff meeting, Mrs. Porter discussed the losses incurred when employees take small items for personal use. What other employee behaviors can result in losses for a health care facility?

_____

_____

_____

_____

9. What do you think about Dee's statement that doctors and supervisors who make a lot of money shouldn't worry about employees taking a few supplies?

_____

_____

_____

_____

10. The patient at the busy clinic stated that the nurses made her feel unimportant. What could they have done differently, even though they were understaffed and behind schedule?

_____

_____

_____

_____

11. Eileen said she didn't realize that patient confidentiality applied to her conversations with her family. What other mistakes might be easy for health care workers to make regarding patient confidentiality?

_____

_____

_____

_____

12. What are some possible legal consequences of breaking patient confidentiality?

_____

_____

_____

_____

CLASS ACTIVITIES

Class Activity 4-1: Medical Ethics Over the Centuries

The Oath of Hippocrates

I swear by Apollo Physician and Aesculapius and Hygeia and Panacea and all the gods and goddesses, making them my witnesses, that I will fulfill according to my ability and judgment this oath and this covenant:

To hold him who has taught me this art as equal to my parents and to live my life in partnership with him, and if he is in need of money to give him a share of mine, and to regard his offspring as equal to my brothers in male lineage and to teach them this art—if they desire to learn it—without fee and covenant; to give a share of precepts and oral instruction and all the other learning to my sons and to the sons of him who has instructed me and to pupils who have signed the covenant and have taken an other according to the medical law, but to no one else.

I will apply dietetic measures for the benefit of the sick according to my ability and judgment; I will keep them from harm and injustice.

I will neither give a deadly drug to anybody if asked for it nor will I make a suggestion to this effect. Similarly, I will not give to a woman an abortive remedy. In purity and holiness I will guard my life and my art.

I will not use the knife, not even on sufferers from stone, but will withdraw in favor of such men as are engaged in this work.

Whatever houses I may visit, I will come for the benefit of the sick, remaining free of all intentional injustice, of all mischief, and in particular of sexual relations with both female and male persons, be they free or slaves.

Source: Lindh, W., Pooler, M., Tamparo, C., & Cerrato, J. (2002). *Delmar's comprehensive medical assisting: Administrative and clinical competencies* (2nd ed.). Clifton Park, NY: Thomson Delmar Learning.

Class Activity 4-2: Ethical Case Studies

Case Study 1

Claudia, a nursing student working in pediatrics, notices that a close family friend whom she has known since childhood has been admitted to the surgery unit. During her lunch break, Claudia quickly reviews his medical record before dropping in to visit him.

- Did Claudia act appropriately? Explain.

Case Study 2

Jaime is a respiratory therapist. One of his patients tells him she needs to confide in someone. She asks him to swear himself to secrecy and then tells him she is feeling very depressed and is thinking about committing suicide after she returns home from the hospital.

- What should Jaime do with this information?

Case Study 3

Catherine is a medical assistant for a cardiologist. She recognizes one of the physician's patients, Mrs. Donnelly, because she is a bus driver for the local school that Catherine's children attend. Mrs. Donnelly has a condition that puts her at risk for a heart attack. She asks Catherine not to report her condition to the bus company because she is afraid she will lose her job and she is a single mother working to put her two sons through college.

- What should Catherine do?

Case Study 4

Cheryl, a medical biller with access to patient charts, notices that a young man who lives in her apartment complex has tested positive for HIV. She wonders whether she should tell the apartment manager that someone with a serious infectious disease is living there.

- What should Cheryl do?

Source for Case Studies 1–4: Adapted from Edge, R., & Groves, J. (1999). *Ethics of health care: A guide for clinical practice.* Clifton Park, NY: Thomson Delmar Learning.

Case Study 5

Jan is a nurse for a gynecologist. Carla, a fifteen-year-old who is a friend of Jan's family, comes to the office for contraceptives. Carla's mother finds the appointment card on her daughter's dresser and calls to find out why Carla was seeing the doctor.

- What should Jan say?
- What determines what she can say to Carla's mother?

Source: Adapted from Haroun, L., & Royce, S. (2004). *Teaching ideas & classroom activities for health care.* Clifton Park, NY: Thomson Delmar Learning.

Case Study 6

Craig is a radiologic technologist who is taking x-rays of an elderly patient for a possible fractured arm. The patient, Mrs. Darnell, seems a bit confused, but seems to be trying to communicate that her family has been "mean" and sometimes hits her.

- What should Craig do?

ASSIGNMENTS

Worksheet for Assignment 4-1: Professional Code of Ethics

Locate and read the professional code of ethics for your occupation. Then answer the following questions:

1. What are the basic underlying principles included in the code?

   _____

   _____

   _____

   _____

   _____

2. List the three guidelines you believe are the most important.

   _____

   _____

   _____

   _____

   _____

3. How might you use the code to guide your future work?

   _____

   _____

   _____

   _____

   _____

Assignment 4-2: Scope of Practice

Locate and read the state practice acts for your occupation. Then complete the following worksheet:

1. List or summarize the tasks and procedures you can perform.

   _____

   _____

   _____

   _____

2. List or summarize the tasks and procedures you are not allowed to perform.

   _____

   _____

   _____

   _____

3. Describe the type of supervision required for your occupational title.

_____

_____

_____

Worksheet for Assignment 4-3: The Cost of Employee Theft

1. BeWell Healthcare has 1,250 employees whose average rate of pay is $15 per hour. If each employee is five minutes late to work once a week for a year, how much money has BeWell lost in wages paid for nonproductive time? (Assume that each employee works 49 weeks per year.) _____

_____

2. If BeWell pays 30 cents each for pens, and each of the 1,250 employees takes home two pens each month, how much will BeWell spend a year for lost pens? _____

_____

3. If 300 of the employees make four personal long-distance calls a year at work that average a cost of $2.80, how much does BeWell spend for its employees' personal calls in a year? _____

_____

_____

4. The total cost to BeWell of these three examples is _____.

5. What other types of loss due to employee actions do you think BeWell might expect? Search the Internet to learn more about the costs of employee theft.

_____

_____

_____

_____

_____

SUGGESTED TOPICS FOR WEB SEARCHES

Ethics

Health care ethics

Medical ethics

Medical malpractice

Medical privacy (HIPAA)

Patient confidentiality

Worksheet for Web Search

Topic: _____

Web address: _____

Sponsoring organization: _____

What I learned: _____

_____

_____

_____

_____

How I might apply what I learned to my work in health care: _____

_____

_____

_____

_____

Name _____ Date _____ Class _____

PRETEST FOR CAREER SUCCESS DVD 4

Select the answer that best completes the sentence, answers the question, or describes the situation.

1. Professional ethics.
   a. are the same as state laws.
   b. are the same for every profession.
   c. are guidelines for employee actions.
   d. are the same as etiquette.

2. When a patient calls the office for test results,
   a. you may not give the information unless the physician gives you permission.
   b. it is okay to give the information if the results are normal.
   c. it is okay to give the information if you are a friend or family member of the patient.
   d. you are never allowed to give test results over the phone.

3. You are asked by your physician to perform a simple test you have not been trained to do. You are uncomfortable about performing the test, but the doctor reassures you and tells you to do it. You should
   a. ask your supervisor for help.
   b. refuse to do the test.
   c. go ahead and do what the doctor has asked you to do.
   d. look in the office procedure manual for instructions.

4. The following are considered part of professional ethics:
   a. the medical assisting scope of practice
   b. good habits of reliability (such as getting to work and returning from breaks on time)
   c. the laws about confidentiality
   d. doing favors for your supervisor

5. The general meaning of "doing the right thing"
   a. is a set of principles that guides professional behavior.
   b. is determined by one's religion, ethnic background, and personal views on ethics.
   c. is always governed by the law.
   d. is usually easy to understand in health care situations.

Circle T if the statement is true or F if the statement is false.

6. T F Many difficult situations in health care make it important for health care workers to have a complete understanding of their professional ethics.

7. T F It is okay to take some office ibuprofen (Advil) when you have a headache at work.

8. T F Health care laws are specific so it is easy for health care workers to decide how to act in every situation.

9. T F In many cases, your own personal code of ethics will give you the means to be a successful health care worker.

10. T F If you are unsure at work, you should ask for assistance.

Name _____ Date _____ Class _____

POSTTEST FOR CAREER SUCCESS DVD 4

Select the answer that best completes the sentence, answers the question, or describes the situation.

1. Health care organizations develop statements of professional ethics

   a. that match health care laws.

   b. to provide the highest-quality service to patients.

   c. to guide the scope of practice of employees.

   d. to encourage employees to get along.

2. The right choice for health care workers to make

   a. is not always the obvious choice.

   b. is easy if the worker follows the employee manual.

   c. is always dictated by laws governing health care.

   d. is easy if you have a good supervisor.

3. Maria's best friend, Jennifer, has come to the office for a pregnancy test. Jennifer is very anxious about the results of the test and she has asked Maria to give her the result. Maria should

   a. give Jennifer the test results. After all, it's just a pregnancy test, not a test for some disease or condition.

   b. refer Jennifer to the physician or nurse as the office policy dictates.

   c. call Jennifer's cell phone and leave a message with the test results in her voice mail.

   d. make a copy of the chart note on the medical record and give it to Jennifer.

4. Your family is visiting from out of town and you decide to go to a local amusement park with them. You did not make arrangements ahead of time, so you call in sick. This is

   a. okay because you have never missed work in the past, so this one time won't hurt.

   b. against employment laws.

   c. a breach of professional ethics.

   d. okay if your employer has been unfair about giving you time off.

5. You are changing out of your uniform after work and find that you have accidentally left a couple of work pens in your pocket. You should

   a. not worry about it because the pens are not really worth much and there are a lot more of them at work.

   b. mention it to your supervisor the next day and apologize.

   c. take the pens back to work the next day.

   d. keep the pens because you feel you've earned them.

6. You have gone out to lunch with a few coworkers. No one is really watching the time, so you go over your one-hour lunch break. This is

   a. a breach of professional ethics.

   b. not a problem because there are only a few patients scheduled this afternoon.

   c. against employment law.

   d. not a problem if your supervisor is with you.

7. You are a medical assistant and your physician has asked you to give a medication that must be given intravenously. This is not included in your scope of practice. What should you do?

   a. Give the medication because it is ordered by the doctor.

   b. Say nothing and ignore the order.

   c. Ask the RN in the office to give the medication.

   d. Tell the doctor he is wrong to ask you to give the medication.

8. To help you always do what is right, you should

   a. know your responsibilities.

   b. always ask the office nurse before performing tests ordered by the doctor.

   c. ask a lot of questions each day.

   d. only do exactly what you are directed to do.

9. When the office is short-staffed and very busy, you should

   a. be courteous to all of your patients and coworkers.

   b. work as quickly as you can, even if it means being a little short with the patients and coworkers at times.

   c. be sure to continue to be nice to patients, but not worry about how you interact with your coworkers.

   d. just keep quiet and work as fast as you can.

10. The experienced nurse in the busy clinic was giving an injection at an angle that was different from the method learned by the new nurse. The new nurse should

   a. correct the nurse as was shown in the scene.

   b. ignore what is happening.

   c. express her concern in private.

   d. tell the doctor she doesn't think the other nurse is competent.

Circle T if the statement is true or F if the statement is false.

11. T F Ethics and laws are the same thing.

12. T F It is important that all health care workers have a complete understanding of their professional ethics.

13. T F Professional ethics are your highest priority.

14. T F It is okay to give results for minor tests to a patient who is a family member or friend.

15. T F It is okay to take sample antibiotics from the office when you have an infection that needs treatment.

Choosing from the list, write the word that corresponds to each definition.

accountability	ampule	compromising
condescending	confidentiality	curt
immense	integrity	professional ethics

_____ 16. Not sharing information

_____ 17. Weakening or giving up something

_____ 18. Treating someone without regard for his or her dignity

_____ 19. Responsibility

_____ 20. Short or brief

_____ 21. A small, sealed container holding a liquid

_____ 22. Very large

_____ 23. Doing what is right and honest

_____ 24. A set of principles that guides a group's decision making regarding what is right and wrong.

DVD 5 PROFESSIONALISM FOR THE HEALTH CARE WORKER

LEARNING OBJECTIVES

1. Understand the importance of professionalism in health care
2. Describe behaviors that demonstrate professionalism
3. Explain how the way you present yourself, including personal hygiene, appearance, and use of language, communicates professionalism

GLOSSARY

burdensome   Difficult to deal with, troublesome.

competence   Level of ability.

continuing education   Classes and training designed to keep professional knowledge and skills up-to-date.

initiative   Taking responsibility for starting or doing something without being told.

perception   One's view of a situation or person.

proactive   Looking for ways to make a positive contribution.

professionalism   A combination of good technical skills, positive attitude, and behaviors that meet certain standards.

reputation   Estimation or opinion about someone or something.

seniority   Priority earned by length of time at a job.

technical competence   Being good at the technical skills required for your job, such as taking vital signs and performing lab tests.

vulnerable   Open to injury or hurt.

DISCUSSION QUESTIONS THAT APPEAR IN DVD 5

Scenes 1 and 2

- Did either Jana or Paula act unprofessionally?

  _____

  _____

- What were the results of their behavior?

  _____

  _____

■ How could they have demonstrated professionalism in their interactions with the patients?

_____

_____

Scene 3

■ Is Shelly wrong in her feelings about her job?

_____

_____

■ What kinds of things could she have done to make her manager more likely to promote her?

_____

_____

Scene 4

■ Why do you think the administration decided a committee was needed to come up with a dress code?

_____

_____

■ Why might some clients feel uncomfortable with health care workers who have tattoos, piercings, and other "modern" fashion trends?

_____

_____

ADDITIONAL DISCUSSION QUESTIONS AND ESSAY PROMPTS

1. "Health care workers provide important services to people when they are at their most vulnerable." What does it mean to be "vulnerable"? What implications does this have for the actions of health care workers?

_____

_____

_____

_____

2. "Patients must feel good about the care they receive." What does this statement mean? Why is more than technical competence needed for patients to feel satisfied?

_____

_____

_____

3. "Beliefs are based on perception." What does this mean? How does it relate to professional appearance and behavior?

_____

_____

_____

_____

4. Jana may be the competent phlebotomist she thinks she is. Why is Sandra concerned about medical mistakes?

_____

_____

_____

_____

5. Think about a negative encounter you have had with an employee of a store or other organization. Did this affect your opinion of the organization? If it did, explain how it influenced your opinion.

_____

_____

_____

_____

6. Both Jana, the phlebotomist, and Paula, the occupational therapist, believe they demonstrate professionalism on the job. Do you think their beliefs are correct? How would you explain to them how others actually perceive them?

_____

_____

_____

_____

7. Do you believe employees should strive for excellence or simply do enough to get by? What should determine how employees are promoted?

_____

_____

_____

_____

8. Shelly believes she is more qualified than Rachel because she has almost three more years of work experience with the company. Do you agree with her? Explain why or why not.

_____

_____

_____

_____

9. What does Mrs. Hastings mean when she says that "the level of professionalism required to get ahead means an employee is proactive"?

_____

_____

_____

10. "Many patients judge your competence by how you look." What does this mean for the health care worker?

_____

_____

_____

11. Describe some of the personal and patient safety issues for health care workers related to their dress, accessories, and hairstyles.

_____

_____

_____

12. How do you feel about having to follow appearance guidelines on the job? What kinds of rules do you find reasonable?

_____

_____

_____

_____

ASSIGNMENTS

Worksheet for Assignment 5-1: Creating Patient Trust

In this segment, the host states that "professionalism means acting in a way that creates patient trust in both you and the organization you work for." Think about the actions of the health care workers in the scenes and answer the following questions:

1. In Scene 1, how did Mandy demonstrate professionalism in her encounter with Sandra?

_____

_____

2. In Scene 1, what did Jana say and do that made Sandra concerned about the quality of care she was receiving?

_____

_____

_____

3. In Scene 2, how did Paula's words and actions plant doubt in Mr. Franklin's mind about the quality of care he was receiving?

_____

_____

_____

4. In Scene 3, what prevented Shelly from being promoted to billing supervisor?

_____

_____

_____

5. In Scene 3, what did Shelly say and do during her conversation to cause Mrs. Hastings to believe that she still did not understand what it takes to receive a promotion?

_____

_____

_____

6. In Scene 4, Paula argues that people should not be judged by their appearance. How might this attitude cause problems with her patients?

_____

_____

_____

Worksheet for Assignment 5-2: Turning It Around

A positive attitude is an important aspect of professionalism. In DVD 5, negativity affects the behavior of several characters. Using the worksheet, suggest ways a positive approach could have improved the outcomes for both the health care workers and their patients.

1. In Scene 1, Sandra suggests that Jana's job might help her get through her personal difficulties. How could Jana be more positive and take advantage of her job to help her?

_____

_____

_____

2. Contrast how Sandra and Jana are dealing with their personal problems.

_____

_____

_____

3. What could Paula, the occupational therapist who is frustrated with the administration at Happy Home Care, do to try to improve her situation?

_____

_____

_____

4. What could Shelly, the medical biller who did not receive the promotion, do to improve her chances of getting promoted?

_____

_____

_____

5. Each of these examples involves the health care worker's attitude. How does attitude affect our actions, both positively and negatively?

_____

_____

_____

Worksheet for Assignment 5-3: How Do You Rate?

Use the worksheet below to rate yourself on some of the important components of professionalism. Think about each statement and check the box you believe best describes your work behavior. Then write goals for any areas you want to improve.

Professional Behavior	Frequently	Usually	Sometimes	Rarely
I am committed to doing my best for future patients and employers.				
Goal(s) for improvement:				
I want to make a positive contribution to the organization for which I work.				
Goal(s) for improvement:				
I view problems as opportunities to learn and make a positive difference.				
Goal(s) for improvement:				
I am willing to leave my personal problems aside and focus on the needs of patients.				
Goal(s) for improvement:				

Professional Behavior	Frequently	Usually	Sometimes	Rarely
Others can count on me to be on time and complete my work.				
Goal(s) for improvement:				
I am willing to follow the rules and policies of my employer, even if I disagree with them.				
Goal(s) for improvement:				
I am willing to represent my employer in a positive light, even if I disagree with policies or procedures.				
Goal(s) for improvement:				

SUGGESTED TOPICS FOR WEB SEARCHES

Customer service

Effect of appearance on patient confidence

Patient satisfaction

Professionalism in health care

Worksheet for Web Search

Topic: _____

Web address: _____

Sponsoring organization: _____

What I learned: _____

_____

_____

_____

How I might apply what I learned to my work in health care: _____

_____

_____

_____

_____

Name _____ Date _____ Class _____

PRETEST FOR CAREER SUCCESS DVD 5

Select the answer that best completes the sentence, answers the question, or describes the situation.

1. Having the skill to successfully practice your occupation is a component of
   a. ethics.
   b. confidentiality.
   c. professionalism.
   d. etiquette.

2. An appropriate way to develop a good relationship with your patient is to
   a. share some personal information with the patient.
   b. be attentive and practice active listening skills.
   c. be as efficient at your job as possible.
   d. ask the patient lots of personal questions.

3. Using poor grammar on the job
   a. won't even be noticed by most patients.
   b. shows poor professionalism.
   c. may be noticed, but really doesn't matter.
   d. is against professional ethics.

4. Looking professional means
   a. always being neat, clean, and well groomed, and wearing the appropriate uniform.
   b. just wearing your uniform each day.
   c. wearing a suit to work each day.
   d. always wearing a smile on your face.

5. Chipped nail polish and dirty shoes
   a. really don't matter to anyone, as long as you do a good job.
   b. are okay as long as your uniform is neat and tidy.
   c. may give the impression of uncleanness.
   d. have no effect on most patients.

Circle T if the statement is true or F if the statement is false.

6. T F Professionalism refers only to technical competence.

7. T F Good grooming is part of professionalism.

8. T F Professionalism goes beyond your work with patients.

9. T F Language and grammar are not part of professionalism, because most patients have poor grammar skills and won't notice your grammar errors.

10. T F Making a positive contribution to the team is a sign of professionalism.

Name _____ Date _____ Class _____

POSTTEST FOR CAREER SUCCESS DVD 5

Select the answer that best completes the sentence, answers the question, or describes the situation.

1. Negative attitude and behavior on the job
   a. can cause patients to doubt the quality of care they are receiving.
   b. are unprofessional.
   c. don't matter as long as you do your tasks well.
   d. are a and b.

2. Professionalism
   a. means acting in a way that creates patient trust in you and the facility you work for.
   b. is only required at hospitals and large clinics.
   c. is how you act around your supervisor.
   d. means getting high grades in your health care classes.

3. Being competent at what you do
   a. is all that is required on the job.
   b. reassures patients, even if your attitude is a little negative.
   c. is only part of what is required to be a true professional.
   d. is not too important if you are part of a large health care team.

4. Shelly is disappointed when she does not get promoted. To be considered for the next promotion, Shelly should
   a. just stop complaining and do her job.
   b. show initiative on the job.
   c. talk to her supervisor's boss.
   d. threaten to quit if she doesn't get promoted.

5. Because she was disappointed that she did not get the promotion, Shelly spoke with her supervisor.
   a. Her behavior was inappropriate. Shelly should have just let it go.
   b. She should have spoken with her supervisor's boss.
   c. She did the professional thing when she spoke to her supervisor.
   d. She should have started looking for another job.

6. The most important reason for wearing long hair pulled back is
   a. you don't want it touching the client's food, wounds, etc.
   b. it's a more conservative look.
   c. this is what employers want.
   d. it looks neater.

7. Jana spoke about her personal problems while she was taking Sandy's blood. Her behavior was

   a. professional because she was efficiently doing the blood draw.

   b. professional because she was developing rapport with the patient by sharing something personal.

   c. unprofessional.

   d. okay because she was just trying to distract Sandy.

8. In one scene, Paula complains to Mr. Franklin about the traffic and the way her manager schedules her day. As a professional, Paula should have

   a. quit her job and found one she was happier with.

   b. spoken to her supervisor and tried to help the company set up a better schedule.

   c. done the best job she could and kept her frustration to herself.

   d. contacted her supervisor's boss about the scheduling issue.

9. Being proactive means

   a. looking for ways to help others without waiting to be told what to do.

   b. doing your job quickly and efficiently.

   c. being cheerful while on the job.

   d. following instructions carefully.

10. Good appearance

    a. will help you create and maintain a positive impression.

    b. is a powerful way to "show what you know."

    c. is part of being a professional.

    d. is all of the above.

Circle T if the statement is true or F if the statement is false.

11. T F Professionalism helps patients feel good about the care they receive.

12. T F Poor grammar is rarely noticed by some patients.

13. T F Positive attitude is a part of professionalism.

14. T F As long as you are in uniform, the rest of your appearance is not important.

15. T F Being a professional is simply about how you work with your patients.

Choosing from the list, write the word that corresponds to each definition

| burdensome | competence | initiative | perception |
| proactive | reputation | technical competence | vulnerable |

_____ 16. Being good at the hands-on skills required for your job

_____ 17. Level of ability

_____ 18. Open to injury or hurt

_____ 19. Difficult to deal with, troublesome

_____ 20. One's view of a situation or person

_____ 21. Estimation or opinion about someone or something

_____ 22. Taking responsibility for starting or doing something without being told

_____ 23. Looking for ways to make a positive contribution

DVD 6   GETTING A JOB IN HEALTH CARE

LEARNING OBJECTIVES

1. Understand the importance of good organization and preparation when conducting your job search
2. Know how to present yourself effectively to potential employers
3. Develop good interviewing skills

GLOSSARY

articulate   To speak clearly.
compassionate   A feeling of wanting to help someone.
genuine   Real, not phony.
initiative   Taking responsibility for starting or doing something without being told.
networking   Letting people know you are looking for work.
pediatric   Dealing with children.
persistence   Keeping at it, not giving up.

DISCUSSION QUESTIONS THAT APPEAR IN DVD 6

Scene 1

■ How would better organization skills have helped Carl in this situation?

_____

_____

■ What types of things should Carl have done to prepare for this job interview?

_____

_____

■ What are some other things that Carl could have done to improve his chances of getting this job?

_____

_____

Scene 2

■ How did Dan present himself during the interview?

_____

_____

- How did Dan's personal appearance make him seem unprofessional?

  _____

  _____

- What are some things that Dan could have talked about to better present his qualifications for the job?

  _____

  _____

Scene 3

- Did Robin demonstrate good interviewing skills?

  _____

  _____

- How did she use examples to present herself?

  _____

  _____

- In what ways did Robin exercise good listening skills during this interview?

  _____

  _____

ADDITIONAL DISCUSSION QUESTIONS AND ESSAY PROMPTS

1. "It has been said that getting a job is a full-time job in itself." Do you agree with this statement? Discuss why or why not.

   _____

   _____

   _____

   _____

2. Networking is an important part of the job search. What is networking and what is the best way to go about it?

   _____

   _____

   _____

   _____

3. Writing thank-you notes is also part of the job search. To whom should you write thank-you notes? What should be included in these notes?

   _____

   _____

   _____

   _____

4. The first applicant is late for his appointment with Mrs. Porter. Why is this one of the most serious mistakes a job applicant can make?

_____

_____

_____

5. Why is it important to learn about a potential employer before attending a job interview?

_____

_____

_____

6. Why is good eye contact important when meeting and speaking with potential employers?

_____

_____

_____

7. Why should job applicants avoid saying negative things about previous employers?

_____

_____

_____

8. What are some ways to learn about a potential employer?

_____

_____

_____

9. When Mrs. Porter asks Dan what he enjoyed most about his training, he responds that he enjoyed doing vital signs because "they were pretty easy to learn." What do you think about this answer?

_____

_____

_____

10. Dan says that he's willing to do his part on the work team as long as the other team members are doing their part. What do you think about his attitude?

_____

_____

_____

11. Dan, the second job applicant, says he thinks passing his medical assisting classes and earning his certificate should be enough to qualify him for a job. Explain why you agree or disagree with his statement.

_____

_____

_____

_____

12. "Employers want to hire people they like." What do you think this means? How should it influence the way you present yourself at a job interview?

_____

_____

_____

_____

13. "Use what the employer tells you to let him or her know how you can contribute to their team." What does this mean? How can you use what you hear to help you in an interview?

_____

_____

_____

_____

14. Will Rogers, an American humorist, said, "You never get a second chance to make a good first impression." How does this relate to a job interview?

_____

_____

_____

_____

CLASS ACTIVITIES

Class Activity Worksheet 6-1: How Should I Answer That?

Here is a list of commonly asked interview questions. Think about how you might answer each one, including examples to demonstrate your skills and characteristics.

1. Tell me something about yourself.

_____

_____

2. Why do you want to work here?

_____

_____

3. How well do you work with others?

_____

_____

_____

4. Which classes did you enjoy the most during your training?

_____

_____

_____

5. How do you handle stress?

_____

_____

_____

6. What procedures and tests can you perform?

_____

_____

_____

7. What other types of jobs have you held?

_____

_____

_____

8. Describe a problem you've had in the workplace and how you handled it.

_____

_____

_____

9. What are you best at?

_____

_____

_____

10. In what areas do you need improvement?

_____

_____

_____

11. What do you believe is the role of customer service in health care?

_____

_____

_____

12. What are your long-term employment goals?

_____

_____

_____

13. Tell me what you know about the equipment you would be using on this job.

_____

_____

_____

ASSIGNMENTS

Worksheet for Assignment 6-1: Keys to a Successful Job Search

Four keys to a successful job search are presented by the host in DVD 6. Describe how each of the three job applicants either did or did not follow these guidelines.

Key 1: Be Prepared

Carl, the first applicant _____

_____

Dan, the second applicant _____

_____

Robin, the third applicant _____

_____

Key 2: Know Yourself

Carl, the first applicant _____

_____

Dan, the second applicant _____

_____

Robin, the third applicant _____

_____

Key 3 : Know the Employer

Carl, the first applicant _____

_____

Dan, the second applicant _____

_____

Robin, the third applicant _____

_____

Key 4: Present Yourself Well

Carl, the first applicant _____

_____

Dan, the second applicant _____

_____

Robin, the third applicant _____

_____

Worksheet for Assignment 6-2: Applying the Keys to a Successful Job Search

Use this worksheet to develop a personal plan for applying each of the success keys.

Key # 1: Be Prepared

My plan _____

_____

_____

_____

Key # 2: Know Yourself

My plan _____

_____

_____

_____

Key # 3: Know the Employer

My plan _____

_____

_____

_____

Key # 4: Present Yourself Well

My plan _____

_____

_____

_____

Worksheet for Assignment 6-3: Researching Potential Employers

Learning about potential employers enables you to see whether a job might be suitable for you, to demonstrate initiative and interest at the interview, and to learn about the employer's needs and how you can best contribute to the organization.

Choose a local health care employer and conduct research to learn as much as you can, using the following questions as a guide.

What type of facility is it? _____

What is the medical specialty (or type of dentistry, or billing services, etc.)? _____

_____

How many employees work there? _____

What type of patients are served? _____

What is the mission of the organization? _____

_____

How can prospective employees learn more? _____

_____

Other information: _____

_____

_____

_____

_____

Worksheet for Assignment 6-4: What Do I Have to Offer?

Use the Worksheet for Assignment 6-4 to begin an inventory of your technical skills, professional competencies, and related work experiences, including examples for each. Technical skills include things like performing tests, taking vital signs, and doing insurance coding. Professional competencies are things like being dependable, being on time, and working well with others.

Technical Skills Related to My Occupational Area	Examples I Can Use
1.	
2.	
3.	
4.	
5.	
6.	
7.	
8.	
9.	
10.	

Professional Competencies	Examples I Can Use
1.	
2.	
3.	
4.	
5.	
6.	
7.	
8.	
9.	
10.	
Experiences, Either at Work or Personal, That Relate to a Job in Health Care	Description of the Experience
1.	
2.	
3.	
4.	
5.	
6.	
7.	
8.	
9.	
10.	

Worksheet for Assignment 6-5: What Can I Ask?

Being prepared to ask questions in an interview helps you learn what is important to the employer. It also shows the employer that you are interested in the job and have taken the time to think about it. Use the Worksheet for Assignment 6-5 and write ten questions you might ask at an interview.

1. _____
   _____

2. _____
   _____

3. _____
   _____

4. _____
   _____

5. _____
   _____

6. _____
   _____

7. _____
   _____

8. _____
   _____

9. _____
   _____

10. _____
    _____

SUGGESTED TOPICS FOR WEB SEARCHES

Health care careers

Interviewing skills

Job search skills

Questions to ask at interviews

Worksheet for Web Search

Topic: _____

Web address: _____

Sponsoring organization: _____

What I learned: _____

_____

_____

_____

_____

How I might apply what I learned to my job search: _____

_____

_____

_____

_____

Name _____ Date _____ Class _____

PRETEST FOR CAREER SUCCESS DVD 6

Select the answer that best completes the sentence, answers the question, or describes the situation.

1. The very first step in getting a job is
   a. setting up the interview.
   b. talking to the placement department at school.
   c. getting yourself organized.
   d. calling employers for information.

2. An important part of advance preparation for interviewing is
   a. making appointments with employers.
   b. having copies of your resume prepared.
   c. discussing it with your placement coordinator.
   d. writing a cover letter.

3. When the interviewer asks you to "Tell me about yourself," the interviewer
   a. wants you to spend a minute or two discussing your skills and how your qualifications fit the employer's needs.
   b. wants you to tell your age and other vital statistics.
   c. wants you to tell how many children you have and your child care arrangements.
   d. is just being friendly and trying to make you feel comfortable.

4. Appropriate dress and grooming for an interview
   a. are not important, as long as you can show you have learned the skills you need to do the job.
   b. are important and demonstrate your level of professionalism.
   c. always include a suit for men and a dress for women.
   d. depend on the job you are applying for.

5. When interviewing, you should
   a. be open and genuine.
   b. answer questions the way you think the interviewer wants you to.
   c. use the shortest answers possible for each question.
   d. talk as much as possible so the interviewer can get to know you better.

Choose T if the statement is true and F if the statement is false.

6. T F   If you have had a previous negative employment experience, you should share it with the interviewer.

7. T F   Good preparation requires anticipating the kinds of questions you might be asked and having some answers prepared.

8. T F   It is not necessary to communicate with the interviewer after the interview.

9. T F   Interviewers won't care if you show up for the interview a few minutes late due to traffic.

10. T F   You should know a little about the employer before you attend an interview.

Name _____ Date _____ Class _____

POSTTEST FOR CAREER SUCCESS DVD 6

Select the answer that best completes the sentence, answers the question, or describes the situation.

1. Preparing for an interview involves

   a. having your clothes and resume ready to go.

   b. having a copy of your grade transcripts to take to the interview.

   c. knowing someone at the organization or office where you will be interviewing.

   d. asking someone at your school to put in a good word for you.

2. In the first scene, Carl showed up for his interview twenty minutes late.

   a. Genevieve Porter is understanding, so being late has had no affect on Carl's chances of getting the job.

   b. This really doesn't matter because Carl has great medical assisting skills.

   c. This is likely to decrease Carl's chances of getting this job.

   d. This is okay because Carl had a good excuse.

3. Dan shows up for his interview poorly groomed.

   a. This doesn't really matter because Dan has excellent medical assisting skills.

   b. This makes Mrs. Porter question Dan's level of professionalism.

   c. This may matter to some interviewers, but not to most.

   d. This is okay because Dan came directly from his current part-time job.

4. Knowing your qualifications

   a. is important so you can present them to a prospective employer.

   b. is not important because they are listed on your resume.

   c. is not important if you have a certificate showing you completed a health care program or earned a degree.

   d. is not important because the employer assumes you are qualified before setting up an interview.

5. During an interview, good listening skills

   a. aren't important because you will be doing most of the talking.

   b. are critical to your success.

   c. won't be noticed by the interviewer.

   d. aren't as important as demonstrating your technical skills.

6. Who was the most successful interviewee in DVD 6?

   a. Carl

   b. Dan

   c. Robin

   d. They were all about equal.

7. Going into an interview, your goal should be
   a. learning as much as you can about this type of office.
   b. learning as much as you can about your future supervisor.
   c. letting the employer know that you can meet his or her needs.
   d. learning more about the job and how much it pays.

8. Enthusiasm and sincerity
   a. are keys to possessing good interviewing skills.
   b. should be toned down during the interview.
   c. matter to some prospective employers, but not to most.
   d. are not important if you have good technical skills.

9. During his interview, Dan spoke about an experience at his last job.
   a. This was a good way to let the interviewer know he has experience.
   b. His response was negative and did not demonstrate good interviewing skills.
   c. This helped him show that he is a team player.
   d. This should not affect the impression Mrs. Porter has of him.

10. During her interview, Robin
    a. was too enthusiastic.
    b. should not have shared the stretching exercise because it had nothing to do with the job.
    c. appeared to be sincere and caring.
    d. was too friendly.

Choose T if the statement is true or F if the statement is false.

11. T F Being a successful job applicant means you get every job you apply for.
12. T F Employers will ask questions only about your work experience.
13. T F Good interviewing skills include using good manners.
14. T F Your answers to interview questions should be what the interviewer wants to hear.
15. T F Your technical skills do not have to be explained if they are listed on your resume.

Choosing from the list, write the word that corresponds to each definition.

| articulate | compassionate | genuine |
| networking | pediatric | persistence |

_____ 16. Keeping at it, not giving up
_____ 17. A feeling of wanting to help someone
_____ 18. Real, not phony
_____ 19. To speak clearly
_____ 20. Dealing with children
_____ 21. Talking with health care professionals about your job search